Essential Oils for First Aid :

A Comprehensive Aromatherapy Guide to Healing

Frances Raven

Contents

Introduction

In a world that thrives on constant progress and modern advancements, there's a quiet resurgence of interest in the age-old wisdom of natural remedies. As we grapple with the fast-paced demands of our lives, we're increasingly drawn to the soothing embrace of nature's bounty, seeking solace and healing in the arms of time-honored traditions. One such tradition that has garnered renewed attention is the use of essential oils as a form of first aid—a practice rooted in centuries of wisdom that is finding a well-deserved place in our modern lives.

From the aromatic gardens of ancient civilizations to the shelves of modern apothecaries, essential oils have traversed time, remaining steadfast in their ability to nurture and heal. This book, *"Essential Oils for First Aid: A Comprehensive Aromatherapy Guide to Healing"* embarks on a journey to explore the intricate relationship between essential oils and the art of first aid. Within these pages, we delve into the origins, science, and practical applications of using essential oils to address a myriad of everyday health concerns.

Unearthing Nature's Bounty

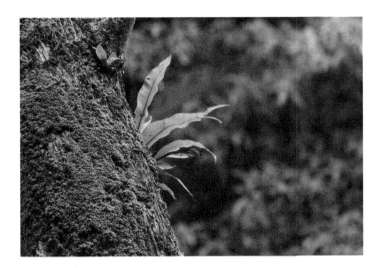

The Aromatic World of Essential Oils: An Intricate Journey of Nature's Essence

In the realm of holistic wellness and natural remedies, essential oils have emerged as powerful and alluring agents that bridge the gap between science and tradition. These aromatic extracts, derived from plants through meticulous processes, possess a myriad of therapeutic and aromatic qualities that have been cherished for centuries across various cultures. The world of essential oils is a captivating tapestry of scents, healing potential, and ancient wisdom, offering a journey into the heart of nature's essence.

A Fragrant History: From Ancient Wisdom to Modern Application

The history of essential oils is entwined with the annals of human civilization, stretching back to ancient times. Early cultures such as the Egyptians, Greeks, and Chinese documented their use of aromatic plants for rituals, medicine, and cosmetics. The Egyptians utilized essential oils for embalming, religious ceremonies, and perfumery, with the precious scents often associated with spirituality and divine connections. Greek scholars like Hippocrates and Dioscorides explored the medicinal properties of plants, laying the foundation for the therapeutic applications of essential oils.

The Middle Ages witnessed the advent of distillation, a process that allowed for the extraction of essential oils in a more refined manner. Avicenna, a Persian physician and philosopher, contributed significantly to the understanding of distillation techniques and the potential benefits of essential oils. As civilizations intertwined through trade routes, essential oils made their way across continents, enriching cultural practices and expanding their global significance.

In modern times, the resurgence of interest in natural remedies and holistic wellness has propelled essential oils into the limelight once again. Their versatile applications, ranging from aromatherapy and personal care to culinary and cleaning purposes, have garnered attention from individuals seeking alternatives to synthetic products. The science behind essential oils has also evolved, with researchers investigating their chemical compositions and physiological effects, further validating their therapeutic potential.

Chapter Two:

Science of Scents: The Art and Science of Extraction

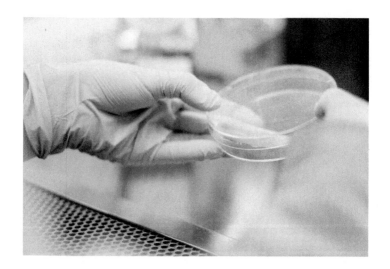

At the heart of essential oils lies the intricate process of extraction, where the very essence of plants is captured. Distillation, steam extraction, cold-pressing, and solvent extraction are among the techniques employed to yield these precious substances. Each method preserves specific compounds and scents, resulting in oils with distinct properties.

The chemical complexity of essential oils is a testament to the multifaceted nature of plants. Compounds such as terpenes, phenols, aldehydes, and esters contribute to their fragrance, flavor, and therapeutic effects. Lavender, for instance, is renowned for its calming aroma and potential to promote relaxation, owing to its high content of linalool and linalyl acetate.

Aromatherapy, a branch of alternative medicine, harnesses the aromatic allure of essential oils to enhance emotional, mental, and physical well-being. The inhalation of these potent scents can influence mood, alleviate stress, and stimulate memory recall. Lavender, chamomile, and bergamot are renowned for their soothing properties, while invigorating oils like peppermint and citrus varieties can uplift and energize.

The application of essential oils extends beyond olfactory stimulation. When diluted and applied topically, some oils possess remarkable skin-soothing and muscle-relaxing effects. Tea tree oil, celebrated for its antibacterial properties, finds utility in skincare routines, while eucalyptus oil's respiratory benefits make it a common ingredient in chest rubs and inhalants.

Embarking on a Aromatic Journey

The world of essential oils is a captivating realm where science harmonizes with ancient wisdom, and nature's gifts intertwine with human innovation. As we delve deeper into this fragrant realm, we discover the nuanced symphony of scents that resonate with our senses and emotions. From the therapeutic embrace of aroma-therapy to the vibrant palette of culinary exploration, essential oils invite us to embark on a journey of holistic well-being and discovery, connecting us to the very essence of the natural world.

Exploring the Versatile Ways of Using Essential Oils

Essential oils have been cherished for centuries due to their aromatic, therapeutic, and even culinary properties. Derived from plants through processes like steam distillation or cold pressing, these potent extracts capture the essence of nature's botanical wonders. The ways of using essential oils are as diverse as their benefits, offering a spectrum of applications that enhance well-being, ambiance, and daily routines.

1. Aromatherapy:
Aromatherapy, the practice of using essential oils to promote physical and psychological well-being, is one of the most well-known applications. Inhaling the aromas of essential oils can have profound effects on emotions, stress levels, and mood. By using a diffuser, steam inhalation, or simply adding a few drops to a tissue or pillow, you can create a serene environment, uplift your spirits, or relax after a long day.

2. Massage and Topical Application:
Applying diluted essential oils to the skin can provide localized benefits. Essential oils can be mixed with carrier oils like coconut, jojoba, or almond oil to create massage blends.

Massaging these blends onto the body not only promotes relaxation but also allows the therapeutic properties of the oils to be absorbed through the skin. This method is commonly used for pain relief, skincare, and muscle relaxation.

3. Bathing and Personal Care:
Adding a few drops of essential oils to your bathwater can turn your bath into a luxurious, aromatic experience. The steam from the bath helps release the aroma, creating a soothing atmosphere. Essential oils can also be incorporated into personal care products like shampoos, conditioners, lotions, and soaps, enhancing their benefits and fragrance.

4. Inhalation and Respiratory Support:
Inhaling essential oils directly from the bottle or through steam inhalation can provide respiratory relief. Eucalyptus, peppermint, and tea tree oils, for instance, have properties that can help clear congestion and soothe irritated airways. This method is particularly useful during cold and allergy seasons.

5. Cleaning and Home Fragrance:
Essential oils offer a natural and aromatic alternative for cleaning and freshening up your living space. Their antimicrobial and antibacterial properties make them effective additions to homemade cleaning solutions. Citrus oils like lemon and orange not only disinfect but also leave a refreshing scent. Additionally, creating DIY room sprays with essential oils can instantly transform the ambiance of your home.

6. Culinary Uses:
Certain essential oils, such as peppermint, lemon, and basil, are safe for culinary use. A single drop of a culinary-grade essential oil can infuse dishes with intense flavors and aromas. These oils are particularly popular in baking, salad dressings, marinades, and beverages.

7. Meditation and Mindfulness:
Using essential oils during meditation and mindfulness practices can deepen your experience. The calming scents of lavender, frankincense, or sandalwood can help create a serene environment conducive to relaxation and self-awareness. Applying oils to pulse points or diffusing them in the meditation space can enhance the soothing effects.

8. Hair and Scalp Health:
Essential oils can address various hair and scalp concerns. Adding a few drops to your shampoo or conditioner can help improve hair texture, manage dandruff, and support a healthy scalp. Massaging diluted oils into the scalp can stimulate blood circulation and promote hair growth.

9. Natural Insect Repellent:
Many essential oils possess natural insect-repelling properties. Oils like citronella, lemongrass, and lavender can be used to create effective and pleasant-smelling insect repellent sprays or balms.

10. Mood Enhancement and Emotional Well-Being:
Essential oils have the power to influence emotions and enhance emotional well-being. Scents like lavender and

chamomile are often used to alleviate stress, anxiety, and even insomnia. Creating personal blends or using oils as part of a self-care routine can have a positive impact on mental health.

Precautions When Using Essential Oils

In our pursuit of nature's remedies, it's crucial to navigate the modern world armed with knowledge. While these oils are gifts from nature, their potency demands respect and informed usage. By understanding the do's and don'ts, readers can ensure that their aromatic journey is both effective and secure.

Dilution: Essential oils are highly concentrated and potent. They should always be diluted with a carrier oil (like coconut or almond oil) before being applied to the skin to avoid irritation.

Avoid Ingestion: Ingesting essential oils can be toxic and should be generally avoided. There are some that can be used in very small quantities though. Even inhaling excessive amounts of undiluted oil can be harmful, causing respiratory distress.

Allergies: Some individuals may be allergic to various essential oils.

It's recommended to perform a patch test before using one extensively.

Children and Pets: Essential oils should be kept out of reach of children and pets, as they can be toxic when ingested or improperly used.

Medical Conditions and Medications: Individuals with certain medical conditions (such as epilepsy or high blood pressure) or those taking specific medications should consult a healthcare professional before using certain essential oils.

In Conclusion:

The ways of using essential oils are as diverse as the oils themselves. Whether through aromatherapy, massage, personal care, cleaning, or culinary adventures, essential oils offer a natural and holistic approach to enhancing various aspects of life. Before incorporating essential oils into your routine, it's important to research their properties, dilution ratios, and any potential contraindications to ensure safe and effective use.

Chapter Three:

The Essential Arsenal:
Must-Have Oils for First Aid

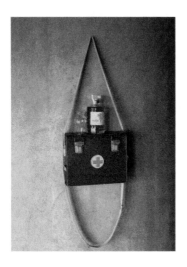

An essential oil first aid kit is a compact and versatile collection of potent natural extracts, designed to provide immediate and holistic solutions for common ailments and injuries. This thoughtfully curated kit combines the healing power of essential oils with the convenience of on-the-go application.

Ideally contained within a compact case, the essential oil first aid kit includes a range of essential oils renowned for their therapeutic properties. Lavender oil, with its soothing and antiseptic qualities, serves as a versatile go-to for cuts, burns, and minor skin irritations. Tea tree oil, a potent antiseptic, aids in treating insect bites, fungal infections, and minor wounds.

Eucalyptus oil, prized for its decongestant and antibacterial effects, offers respiratory relief and can be beneficial for colds and sinus issues. Peppermint oil's cooling sensation helps alleviate headaches, muscle pain, and nausea.

This book will show you that an essential oil kit is not only an must-have companion for outdoor adventures and travel but also an empowering tool to address everyday health concerns naturally and effectively.

Chapter Four:

Tea Tree Oil: Nature's Potent Elixir for Health and Well-Being

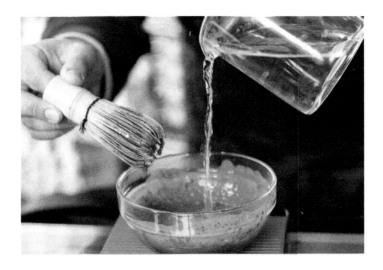

"Tea tree oil is a botanical gem, a testament to nature's ability to nurture and protect."
- Dr. Joseph Mercola

In the vast realm of essential oils, few have garnered as much attention and acclaim as tea tree oil. Derived from the leaves of the Melaleuca alternifolia tree native to Australia, tea tree oil has emerged as a versatile and potent elixir with a plethora of therapeutic benefits. From its indigenous use by Australian Aboriginals to its global popularity today, tea tree oil's remarkable properties have solidified its place in modern natural medicine, skin care, and household applications.

A Glimpse into Tea Tree's Rich History

Tea tree oil's story traces back centuries, deeply rooted in the traditions of the Indigenous people of Australia. The Aboriginals were among the first to recognize the oil's potential, using it for its antiseptic and healing properties. The leaves of the Melaleuca alternifolia tree were crushed and applied topically to wounds, cuts, and infections. This practice showcased the natural antibacterial properties of tea tree oil, fostering its reputation as a valuable natural remedy.

The oil's name, "tea tree," is said to have originated from the 18th-century British explorer Captain James Cook. Upon his voyage to the land Down Under, he observed the locals brewing a tea-like beverage using the leaves of the Melaleuca alternifolia tree. This nomenclature has persisted, despite the fact that tea tree oil is not derived from the same plant as tea leaves.

The Science Behind Tea Tree Oil's Power

The potency of tea tree oil lies in its complex chemical composition, which includes terpinen-4-ol, cineole, and other terpenes. Terpinen-4-ol is considered the primary active ingredient responsible for many of the oil's antimicrobial and antiseptic properties. These properties make tea tree oil an effective tool against various microorganisms, including bacteria, viruses, and fungi.

Research has consistently validated the antimicrobial effects of tea tree oil. Studies have demonstrated its efficacy in treating skin infections, wounds, acne, and even fungal conditions like athlete's foot and nail fungus. Its natural ability to inhibit the growth of harmful microorganisms without harming beneficial ones has led to its application in a wide range of health-related products.

A Versatile Natural Remedy

Tea tree oil's versatility is a hallmark of its popularity. Its applications span across various fields, from holistic health to personal care, and even household cleaning.

In skin care, tea tree oil's potential shines. Its ability to manage acne has garnered significant attention. Its anti-inflammatory properties help soothe redness and irritation associated with acne, while its antibacterial action targets the bacteria that contribute to breakouts. When properly diluted, it can be applied topically as a spot treatment or added to facial cleansers and moisturizers.

Furthermore, tea tree oil's antifungal properties make it an effective treatment for common fungal infections like athlete's foot, yeast infections, and ringworm. Its versatility doesn't stop at the skin; it can be incorporated into shampoos to combat dandruff and promote a healthier scalp.

Tea Tree Oil in Modern Medicine

The journey of tea tree oil from traditional remedy to modern medicine is a testament to its efficacy. Today, it can be found as an ingredient in various over-the-counter products such as creams, ointments, shampoos, and mouthwashes. It has also found a place in dentistry due to its potential in combating oral bacteria, making it a valuable addition to oral hygiene products.

Beyond topical applications, tea tree oil's benefits can extend to aromatherapy. When diffused, its invigorating and earthy scent can help create a calming and revitalizing atmosphere. Inhaling tea tree oil's aroma may also have potential benefits for respiratory health.

A Note on Safety and Proper Usage

While tea tree oil offers numerous benefits, it's important to use it with care and knowledge. Due to its potency, it should always be diluted before being applied to the skin to prevent irritation. A carrier oil, such as coconut oil or jojoba oil, can be used for this purpose. Additionally, some individuals may be sensitive or allergic to tea tree oil, so a patch test is recommended before widespread use.

Ingesting tea tree oil is generally considered unsafe and is not recommended. Its concentration of compounds can be harmful when ingested, and there is limited scientific evidence supporting its internal use. As with any essential oil, pregnant and breastfeeding individuals, as well as those with specific medical conditions, should consult a healthcare professional before using tea tree oil.

Conclusion: Tea Tree Oil's Enduring Legacy

Tea tree oil's journey from ancient indigenous practices to modern-day applications is a captivating tale of nature's potency harnessed by human innovation. Its remarkable antimicrobial, anti-inflammatory, and antifungal properties have positioned it as a staple in the world of holistic health, skin care, and even household cleaning. As we navigate an era marked by a renewed appreciation for natural remedies, tea tree oil's enduring legacy continues to thrive, inviting us to tap into the healing potential of the natural world. With proper understanding and caution, this potent elixir can enhance our well-being and empower us to explore the holistic benefits that nature offers.

Chapter Five:

Lavender Oil: The Essence of Tranquility and Healing

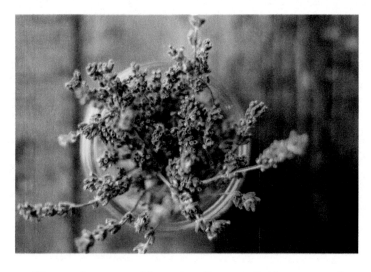

"Lavender, sweet blooming flower of calmness and tranquility, is the messenger of peace."
- Dodinsky

In the world of essential oils, few are as beloved and versatile as lavender oil. Renowned for its soothing aroma and a myriad of therapeutic properties, lavender oil has etched its place in both ancient practices and modern holistic wellness. From the fields of

Provence to the laboratories of aromatherapy, lavender oil's captivating fragrance and diverse applications have solidified its status as an essential element of natural medicine, relaxation, and rejuvenation.

A Blossom of History and Symbolism

Lavender, with its delicate purple flowers and intoxicating scent, has graced gardens, perfumeries, and apothecaries for centuries. Its origins can be traced back to the Mediterranean region, where it was cultivated by ancient civilizations such as the Egyptians, Greeks, and Romans. The Romans, in particular, appreciated lavender for its aromatic allure and believed in its protective and purifying properties.

Throughout history, lavender has been associated with love, purity, and devotion. Its name is derived from the Latin word "lavare," meaning "to wash," highlighting its historical use in bathing and perfumery. In medieval times, lavender was strewn on the floors of homes and castles to ward off unpleasant odors and pests. Its fragrant presence also found its way into sachets, pomanders, and even medical preparations during the plague-ridden years.

The Distillation of Lavender's Essence

The journey to capturing lavender's aromatic essence begins with the process of steam distillation. Lavender flowers are harvested at their peak, and their essential oil is extracted by subjecting them to steam. The steam carries the volatile aromatic compounds from the flowers, and as it condenses, it yields the precious lavender oil.

The resulting oil is a complex composition of constituents, with linalool and linalyl acetate being the primary contributors to its distinct scent and therapeutic effects. These compounds are responsible for lavender oil's calming and relaxing properties, making it a staple in aromatherapy practices.

Aromatherapy: The Power of Lavender's Aroma

One of the most notable applications of lavender oil is in aromatherapy, a practice that harnesses the power of scents to influence mood, emotions, and well-being. Lavender's fragrance is universally recognized for its ability to promote relaxation and calmness. Inhaling the aroma of lavender oil can alleviate stress, anxiety, and restlessness, making it a valuable tool for managing the demands of modern life.

Aromatherapists often diffuse lavender oil in homes, offices, and wellness spaces to create a serene and tranquil atmosphere. It can also be blended with carrier oils and applied topically to pulse points or added to baths for a rejuvenating sensory experience.

A Multitude of Therapeutic Applications

Lavender oil's therapeutic potential extends beyond its calming aroma. Its versatile properties make it a prized ingredient in a wide array of applications, ranging from skin care to first aid.

In skin care, lavender oil's anti-inflammatory and antiseptic properties can benefit a variety of skin conditions. It can be used to soothe minor burns, cuts, and insect bites, promoting healing and reducing discomfort. Its gentle nature also makes it suitable for individuals with sensitive skin, and it is often included in formulations for creams, lotions, and serums.

Lavender oil's ability to promote relaxation has led to its use in sleep-related practices. Adding a few drops to a diffuser before bedtime or incorporating it into a pre-sleep routine can help create a calming ambiance conducive to a restful night's sleep.

Scientific Validation and Modern Application

The efficacy of lavender oil is not solely rooted in tradition; modern research has illuminated its potential benefits. Studies have shown that inhaling lavender oil can lead to a reduction in anxiety levels and improved sleep quality. Its anti-inflammatory and antioxidant properties contribute to its potential role in skin health and wound healing.

In clinical settings, lavender oil has been explored as a complementary therapy for various conditions, including anxiety disorders, postoperative pain, and even dementia-related agitation. While more research is needed to establish its precise mechanisms and applications, these studies underscore lavender oil's potential to bridge the gap between traditional wisdom and evidence-based medicine.

A Note on Safety and Usage

Lavender oil is generally considered safe for topical and inhalation use when properly diluted. However, as with any essential oil, precautions should be taken to avoid adverse reactions. Conducting a patch test prior to widespread application can help identify any sensitivities or allergies. Additionally, using too much undiluted lavender oil on the skin can potentially cause irritation.

Conclusion: Lavender Oil's Lasting Legacy

Lavender oil's timeless allure continues to captivate people across cultures and generations. Its soothing aroma, rich history, and versatile applications have firmly established its role in promoting relaxation, healing, and overall well-being. As we navigate the complexities of modern life, lavender oil serves as a reminder of nature's capacity to provide solace and rejuvenation. Whether enjoyed through the calming embrace of aromatherapy or incorporated into skincare rituals, lavender oil's lasting legacy reminds us of the delicate balance between tradition and innovation in the pursuit of holistic health and tranquility.

Chapter Six:

Eucalyptus Oil: Nature's Gift for Health and Wellness

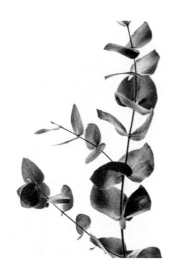

"Eucalyptus oil: a balm for the senses, a sanctuary of clarity amid life's chaos." - Unknown

In the world of natural remedies and essential oils, few hold the remarkable reputation of eucalyptus oil. Derived from the leaves of the eucalyptus tree, this aromatic oil has been utilized for centuries for its myriad health benefits. From respiratory support to its antimicrobial properties, eucalyptus oil has carved a niche for itself in both traditional and modern medicine.

Historical Significance:

Eucalyptus, native to Australia, has been cherished by Indigenous communities for generations. The Aboriginal people used the leaves of the eucalyptus tree to create poultices to treat wounds and alleviate symptoms of respiratory ailments. As European settlers arrived in Australia, they quickly adopted the medicinal properties of eucalyptus, leading to its spread across the world. The oil, extracted through steam distillation, contains potent compounds like eucalyptol, which gives the oil its distinctive scent and therapeutic properties and has a rich history of utilization, dating back centuries, and its versatility continues to amaze researchers, aromatherapists, and manufacturers alike.

Extraction Process:

The process of extracting eucalyptus oil primarily involves steam distillation, a method that harnesses the volatile components of the plant material. Eucalyptus leaves are carefully selected and harvested. The choice of leaves greatly affects the quality of the oil, and factors such as age, health, and aroma play a significant role. The harvested leaves undergo steam distillation, where steam is passed through the plant material. As the steam interacts with the leaves, it breaks down the oil glands, releasing the essential oil. The resulting mixture of steam and oil vapor is then condensed and collected. The collected mixture is allowed to settle, and due to the difference in density, the essential oil separates from the condensed water. The oil is then carefully collected, and any remaining water is removed. To ensure the oil's purity and quality, it undergoes rigorous testing for factors like aroma, chemical composition, and potency. This ensures that the extracted eucalyptus oil meets the desired standards.

Eucalyptus oil's versatility is one of its key attractions. It boasts a range of benefits that cater to various aspects of health and wellness.

Respiratory Support: Perhaps one of the most well-known uses of eucalyptus oil is its ability to support respiratory health. The oil's expectorant and decongestant properties can provide relief from colds, coughs, and sinus congestion. Inhalation of eucalyptus oil vapor is known to clear the airways, making it a popular choice in inhalers, vapor rubs, and steam inhalation therapies.

Anti-Inflammatory: Eucalyptus oil possesses anti-inflammatory properties that make it effective in soothing sore muscles and joints. When diluted and massaged onto the skin or added to bath water, it can provide relief from pain and inflammation, making it a preferred oil for athletes and those suffering from arthritis.

Antimicrobial and Antiseptic: Eucalyptus oil contains compounds that exhibit potent antimicrobial and antiseptic properties. It can be used topically to cleanse wounds and prevent infections. Moreover, its strong aroma is believed to deter insects, making it a natural insect repellent.

Mental Clarity and Relaxation: The invigorating aroma of eucalyptus oil is known to promote mental clarity and alertness. It can be used in aromatherapy to boost concentration and alleviate mental fatigue. Conversely, its calming effects can also help in reducing stress and promoting relaxation.

Hair and Scalp Health: Eucalyptus oil can be added to shampoos and conditioners to promote a healthy scalp. It is believed to stimulate hair follicles, improve circulation, and potentially reduce dandruff.

Skin Care: Eucalyptus oil is included in skincare products for its potential to cleanse and soothe the skin. It's often found in cleansers, lotions, and creams.

Oral Health: Due to its antimicrobial properties, eucalyptus oil is sometimes included in oral hygiene products like toothpaste and mouthwash. It may help combat bacteria responsible for bad breath and plaque buildup.

Fever Reducer: Eucalyptus oil's cooling sensation can help reduce fever when applied topically. Its ability to induce sweating can aid the body in cooling down during a fever.

Industrial and Household Applications:

Eucalyptus oil extends its utility beyond personal care and wellness, finding applications in various industrial and household settings:

Cleaning Products: Due to its antiseptic properties and pleasant fragrance, eucalyptus oil is used as an ingredient in natural cleaning products. It helps disinfect surfaces and freshen indoor environments.

Insect Repellent: Eucalyptus oil serves as a natural insect repellent. When diluted and applied to skin or clothes, it can help deter mosquitoes and other pests.

Flavoring and Fragrance: In the food and beverage industry, eucalyptus oil is occasionally used to add flavor to products like candies and cough drops. It's also employed in perfumes, candles, and air fresheners.

Conclusion:

Eucalyptus oil's journey from ancient traditions to modern wellness practices underscores its enduring value. With its remarkable range of benefits spanning respiratory health, pain relief, and beyond, this essential oil continues to capture the attention of those seeking natural solutions for their well-being. However, responsible use and awareness of precautions are essential to harness its potential without compromising safety. As the world continues to explore the wonders of holistic health, eucalyptus oil remains a timeless companion on this journey toward wellness and sustainable living.

Chapter Seven:

Citronella Oil: A Natural Shield Against Pests and More

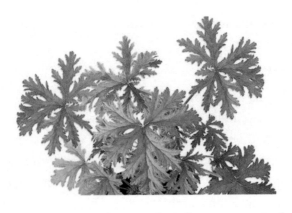

"In the whisper of citronella oil's scent, we find a symphony of nature's defenses harmonizing with our desire for serenity." - Oliver Woods

Few natural substances carry the reputation and recognition that citronella oil does. Renowned for its insect-repelling properties, citronella oil has become a staple in many households, gardens, and outdoor activities. However, its potential goes far beyond being just a pest deterrent. This section explores the history, uses, benefits, and precautions associated with citronella oil.

Historical Roots and Extraction:

Citronella oil is derived from Cymbopogon nardus, a grass native to Southeast Asia. The oil is extracted from the plant's leaves through steam distillation, resulting in a distinctive and refreshing citrusy aroma. Its name is derived from the French word "citronelle," which means "lemon balm."

A Natural Shield Against Pests:

One of the most well-known and valued properties of citronella oil is its ability to repel insects. Its scent acts as a deterrent to mosquitoes, flies, and other bothersome pests, making it a popular choice for outdoor gatherings and camping trips. The oil's effectiveness in warding off mosquitoes is often harnessed in candles, sprays, lotions, and diffusers.

Diverse Uses and Benefits:

While citronella oil is celebrated for its insect-repelling prowess, its versatility extends to various other applications in health and wellness:

Aromatherapy: The invigorating and citrusy aroma of citronella oil can have uplifting effects on mood and mental clarity. Its fragrance is often used in aromatherapy to create an ambiance of freshness and positivity.

Relaxation and Stress Relief: Citronella's aroma, when diffused, can help reduce stress and anxiety. Its scent can contribute to a calming atmosphere that promotes relaxation and balance.

Cleaning and Disinfecting: Citronella oil possesses antimicrobial properties, making it a useful addition to homemade cleaning solutions. Its fresh scent can also help mask unpleasant odors.

Natural Deodorant: The antimicrobial qualities of citronella oil can be harnessed in natural deodorants to combat body odor.

Massage and Pain Relief: When diluted with a carrier oil, citronella oil can be applied topically to soothe sore muscles and provide relief from joint discomfort.

Anti-Inflammatory: Citronella oil's anti-inflammatory properties can aid in reducing inflammation and redness when applied to the skin.

Hair Care: Citronella oil is sometimes added to shampoos to help maintain a healthy scalp and potentially deter lice.

Precautions and Considerations:

As with any essential oil, citronella oil requires careful use and consideration of certain precautions:

Skin Sensitivity: Citronella oil may cause skin irritation or allergic reactions in some individuals. Conduct a patch test before applying it to a larger area of skin.

Dilution: Due to its potency, citronella oil should always be diluted with a carrier oil before being applied to the skin. Using it undiluted can lead to irritation.

Avoid Ingestion: Citronella oil is meant for external use only. Ingesting it can cause adverse reactions and is not recommended.

The Balance Between Natural and Chemical Solutions:

Citronella oil's popularity as an insect repellent has positioned it as a natural alternative to chemical-based products. While chemical solutions can offer effective pest control, they often come with environmental and health concerns. Citronella oil provides a natural, eco-friendly alternative that minimizes exposure to potentially harmful chemicals.

Conclusion:

Citronella oil's journey from its historical roots to its modern uses is a testament to its effectiveness and versatility. As a potent insect repellent, it offers a solution to one of humanity's age-old challenges. Beyond that, its aromatic and therapeutic properties contribute to overall well-being. Whether used in outdoor settings, for aromatherapy, or as a natural remedy, citronella oil continues to hold its place as a valuable tool in the quest for holistic health and a pest-free environment. Through responsible use and an understanding of its benefits and precautions, citronella oil remains a symbol of nature's wisdom harnessed for the betterment of our lives.

Chapter Eight:

Peppermint Oil: Nature's Cooling Balm for Body and Mind

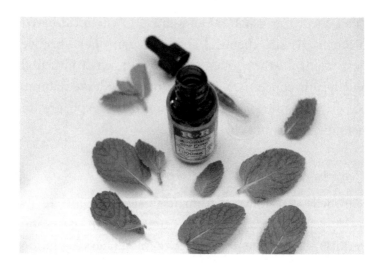

"In the garden of aromas, peppermint oil stands tall, a refreshing testament to nature's brilliance."
- Michael Adams

In the world of essential oils, few possess the remarkable versatility and invigorating properties of peppermint oil. With its distinct aroma, powerful menthol content, and myriad of health benefits, peppermint oil has been cherished for centuries across cultures and traditions. This chapter delves into the history, uses, benefits, and precautions associated with peppermint oil, revealing its multifaceted nature as a natural remedy and aromatic delight.

Aromatic History and Extraction:

Peppermint (Mentha x piperita) is a hybrid plant believed to be a cross between water mint and spearmint. Native to Europe, it has found its way into various corners of the world due to its adaptability and prized qualities. The essential oil is obtained through steam distillation of the leaves, yielding a highly concentrated oil rich in menthol and other active compounds.

An Invigorating Sensation:

Peppermint oil is celebrated for its intense, minty aroma that immediately awakens the senses. This cooling and refreshing fragrance is often associated with feelings of vitality, clarity, and focus. The scent's invigorating qualities have made peppermint oil a staple in aromatherapy, where it is used to stimulate the mind and promote mental alertness.

Versatility in Uses:

Peppermint oil's range of uses spans across various aspects of health and well-being:

Digestive Aid: Peppermint oil is renowned for its ability to support digestion. It can help alleviate symptoms of indigestion, bloating, and gas. Consuming diluted peppermint oil or using it in teas can provide relief from discomfort after meals.

Respiratory Support: The menthol content in peppermint oil contributes to its ability to open up the airways. Inhaling peppermint oil vapor can provide relief from congestion and soothe respiratory discomfort.

Headache Relief: Peppermint oil's cooling properties make it effective in providing relief from headaches. When diluted and applied to the temples or forehead, it can help reduce tension and promote relaxation.

Muscle Relaxant: The soothing effects of peppermint oil on muscles have made it a popular choice for massages. When mixed with a carrier oil and massaged onto sore areas, it can help alleviate muscle tension and discomfort.

Natural Bug Repellent: Peppermint's strong aroma serves as a natural deterrent for insects. A diluted solution of peppermint oil can be used as a bug repellent, providing a chemical-free alternative to commercial products.

Oral Health: The antimicrobial properties of peppermint oil make it a common ingredient in toothpaste, mouthwash, and chewing gum. It can help combat bad breath and promote oral hygiene.

Mind and Mood Enhancement:

The invigorating aroma of peppermint oil has a direct impact on mental clarity and mood. Inhaling its scent can help alleviate mental fatigue, boost concentration, and enhance focus. The cooling sensation it provides can also contribute to a sense of calm and relaxation.

The Intersection of Tradition and Science:

Peppermint oil's long history of use is now backed by scientific research that confirms its various benefits. Its therapeutic qualities have earned it a place not only in traditional practices but also in modern wellness approaches.

Conclusion:

Peppermint oil's journey from its aromatic origins to its versatile applications in health and well-being highlights its unique place in the world of essential oils. With its ability to refresh the mind, soothe the body, and uplift the spirit, peppermint oil is a timeless companion in the quest for holistic wellness. Whether used for digestive support, respiratory relief, or as an invigorating aroma, peppermint oil continues to be a testament to nature's power to enhance our lives. Adhering to precautions and guidelines ensures that this potent oil is harnessed to its fullest potential while maintaining safety. Through centuries of appreciation and continued exploration, peppermint oil remains a fragrant reminder of the natural wonders that contribute to our overall vitality and balance.

Chapter Nine:

Geranium Oil: A Floral Elixir for Balance and Beauty

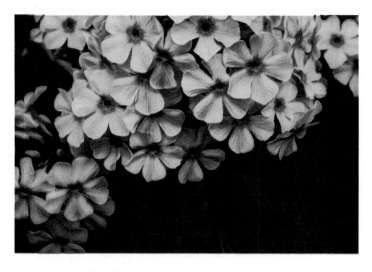

"Geranium oil, with its delicate floral aroma, is nature's way of bringing balance and harmony to the mind and body." - Robert Tisserand

In the essential oil world almost nothing compares with the enchanting allure and therapeutic potential of geranium oil. Derived from the fragrant petals and leaves of the Pelargonium graveolens plant, geranium oil has captivated aromatherapists, beauty enthusiasts, and herbalists for centuries. Its multifaceted aroma, soothing properties, and versatile applications make it a cherished ingredient in various domains, from skincare and wellness to emotional balance and even insect repellency. In this exploration, we embark on a journey through the extraction, historical significance, diverse uses, and potential benefits of geranium oil.

Botanical Beauty:

Geranium oil, also known as Pelargonium oil, is extracted through steam distillation from the leaves and flowers of various Pelargonium species, primarily Pelargonium graveolens. The resulting oil is a concentrated embodiment of the plant's essence.

Native to South Africa, geraniums have found their way into gardens and homes around the world, gracing landscapes with their vibrant blooms and captivating fragrance.

To ensure the purity and authenticity of the oil, rigorous testing is conducted. Aromatherapists and producers assess various factors, including aroma, chemical composition, and potential contaminants, to guarantee the oil's therapeutic efficacy.

Historical and Cultural Significance:

The history of geranium oil is interwoven with various cultures and traditions, each recognizing and harnessing its unique attributes. Ancient Egyptians revered geranium for its aesthetic and aromatic qualities, using it in skincare preparations and perfumes. Throughout history, geranium oil has been celebrated for its potential to balance emotions and promote well-being. Its presence in traditional herbal medicine and folk remedies underscores its enduring popularity.

Diverse Uses and Benefits:

Geranium oil's versatility shines through its wide array of applications, ranging from personal care to emotional support:

Skin Care: Geranium oil's astringent and antiseptic properties make it a valuable asset in skincare. It's often used to address issues such as acne, inflammation, and excessive oiliness. Its rejuvenating properties may also help promote healthy and radiant skin. Geranium oil can help regulate sebum production, making it a valuable addition to skincare routines for both oily and dry skin. It supports optimal hydration without clogging pores.

Anti-Aging: Geranium oil's potential to tighten and tone the skin can reduce the appearance of fine lines and wrinkles, making it a sought-after ingredient in anti-aging products.

Hair Care: When added to shampoos or conditioners, geranium oil can promote a healthy scalp and assist in managing dandruff. Its pleasant aroma is an additional bonus, leaving hair subtly scented.

Balancing the Mind and Emotions:

Geranium oil is celebrated for its ability to restore emotional equilibrium. Its floral scent is both uplifting and calming, making it a staple in aromatherapy practices. Inhaling the aroma of geranium oil can help alleviate stress, anxiety, and even symptoms of depression. Its balancing effect on emotions is believed to stem from its influence on the nervous system, creating a sense of serenity.

Insect Repellent: The aroma of geranium oil acts as a natural deterrent for insects, making it a popular choice for crafting homemade insect repellents. Its ability to keep pesky bugs at bay without the use of harsh chemicals adds to its appeal.

Hormonal Harmony and Women's Health:

Geranium oil's influence extends to women's health by potentially assisting in hormonal balance. It is believed to alleviate menstrual discomfort and symptoms of menopause, offering a natural approach to addressing these transitional phases in a woman's life.

Wound Healing: The antimicrobial and anti-inflammatory properties of geranium oil can accelerate the healing process of wounds, cuts, and minor skin irritations.

Exploring the Intersection of Tradition and Modernity:

Geranium oil's historical significance aligns seamlessly with modern research that validates its therapeutic effects. Its enduring presence in wellness practices highlights its role in enhancing health and well-being.

Conclusion:

Geranium oil's journey from ancient civilizations to modern wellness practices speaks to its timeless appeal and enduring value. Whether used to beautify the skin, balance emotions, or promote women's health, geranium oil offers a fragrant and nurturing experience. Adhering to proper guidelines and precautions ensures its safe and effective use. As the world continues to embrace natural solutions for holistic health, geranium oil remains a fragrant reminder of nature's ability to enhance our lives in both subtle and profound ways. Through the aromatic embrace of geranium oil, we are reminded of the delicate beauty and strength that the natural world offers us, inviting us to embark on a journey of well-being, balance, and self-care.

Chapter Ten:

Chamomile Oil: Nature's Soothing Elixir for Body and Mind

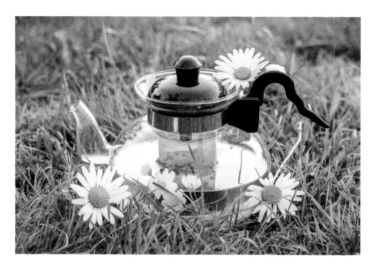

"Chamomile oil: where the sun's warmth and the earth's embrace converge, crafting a fragrant remedy for life's tensions." - Sophia Turner

The gentle yet powerful properties of chamomile oil are virtually unsurpassed. Derived from the flowers of the chamomile plant, this aromatic oil has been revered for centuries for its calming and healing effects. With a history rooted in ancient civilizations and a presence in modern wellness practices, chamomile oil continues to enchant and provide a range of benefits. We explore the history, uses, benefits, and precautions associated with chamomile oil, revealing its comforting embrace for both body and mind.

A Floral Legacy:

Chamomile oil originates from the blossoms of the chamomile plant, belonging to the Asteraceae family. The two most common varieties used for oil extraction are German chamomile (Matricaria chamomilla), which produces a wonderful deep blue oil, and Roman chamomile (Chamaemelum nobile). These delicate flowers, often resembling daisies, hold within them a wealth of therapeutic compounds that have been cherished across cultures and generations.

Ancient Origins and Timeless Wisdom:

Chamomile's use can be traced back to ancient civilizations, where it was revered for its calming properties. The Egyptians dedicated chamomile to their sun god due to the flower's resemblance to the sun's radiant rays. Throughout history, chamomile has been embraced for its ability to soothe the spirit, and its influence extends well into modern times.

Soothing the Senses:

Chamomile oil's gentle aroma is often described as apple like, with hints of earthiness and floral notes. This scent is known for its soothing effect on the mind and emotions. In aromatherapy, chamomile oil is employed to ease anxiety, promote relaxation, and induce restful sleep. Inhaling its delicate aroma can create an atmosphere of tranquility, making it an essential tool for managing stress and finding solace.

A Gift to the Skin:

Chamomile oil's benefits extend to skin care as well:

Skin Calming: Chamomile oil's anti-inflammatory properties make it an effective solution for soothing irritated or sensitive skin. It can alleviate redness, itching, and discomfort caused by conditions like eczema and dermatitis.

Wound Healing: The oil's gentle nature and antimicrobial qualities contribute to its ability to support wound healing and prevent infections.

Acne Relief: Chamomile oil's anti-inflammatory and antibacterial properties make it a valuable addition to skincare routines for those dealing with acne-prone skin.

Anti-aging: Chamomile oil's antioxidants can help protect the skin from damage caused by free radicals, potentially reducing the signs of premature aging.

Digestive Comfort:

Chamomile oil has long been recognized for its benefits in promoting digestive health.

Chamomile oil's carminative properties can help soothe an upset stomach, alleviate gas, and reduce bloating. Its anti-inflammatory and antispasmodic effects are believed to contribute to its potential in relieving symptoms of irritable bowel syndrome (IBS) and other gastrointestinal issues.

Bridging Tradition with Science:

Chamomile oil's journey through time and cultures is now supplemented by scientific research that validates its various benefits. Its continued relevance in wellness practices speaks to its harmonious blend of ancient wisdom and modern understanding.

Conclusion:

Chamomile oil's voyage from ancient rituals to modern wellness practices is a testament to its timeless allure and multifaceted potential. Whether used for its calming effects on the mind, its soothing touch on the skin, or its digestive benefits, chamomile oil offers a gentle embrace of nature's wisdom. Adhering to guidelines and precautions ensures its safe and effective use. Through chamomile oil, we connect with the nurturing power of the natural world, inviting a sense of serenity and rejuvenation into our lives. In the delicate petals of the chamomile flower, we find a reminder of nature's ability to bring comfort and healing to both body and soul.

Chapter Eleven:

Rosemary Oil: A Time-Honored Elixir for Mind and Body

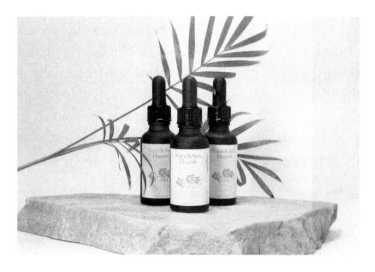

"From memory's embrace to the caress of healthy hair, rosemary oil stands as a testament to nature's capacity to nurture and heal." - Patricia Davis

Rosemary (Rosmarinus officinalis) is an aromatic herb known for its distinctive fragrance and culinary uses. Beyond its role in the kitchen, rosemary has been valued for centuries for its medicinal and therapeutic properties. One of the most popular derivatives of this remarkable herb is rosemary oil, an essential oil that carries with it a plethora of benefits for the mind, body, and spirit. Rosemary oil embodies the resilience and fortitude of its namesake. This plant has earned its place in the annals of herbalism for its ability to thrive in various environments, symbolizing its adaptability and strength.

Historical Significance and Traditional Uses:

The history of rosemary stretches back to ancient civilizations, where it held symbolic and practical importance. The ancient Egyptians used rosemary in their burial rituals to signify remembrance and to honor the departed. The Greeks and Romans believed in its memory-enhancing qualities and used it as a symbol of fidelity and love.

In traditional medicine, rosemary was used for a variety of purposes. It was brewed into teas to aid digestion and alleviate headaches. Its essential oil was also used topically to improve circulation and ease muscle pain. The aromatic leaves were often burned as incense to purify the air and create a calming atmosphere.

Extraction and Composition:

Rosemary oil is extracted through steam distillation from the flowering tops of the rosemary plant. The resulting essential oil contains a complex mixture of chemical compounds, including pinene, camphene, cineole, and borneol. These compounds contribute to the oil's distinctive aroma and therapeutic effects.

The Mind's Awakening:

The invigorating scent of rosemary oil has long been associated with mental clarity and alertness. In aromatherapy, its aroma is known to stimulate cognitive function, boost memory, and enhance focus. Inhaling rosemary oil can elevate mood, reduce mental fatigue, and create an ambiance of revitalization.

Versatility in Uses:

Aromatherapeutic Benefits:

Mental Clarity and Focus: The invigorating scent of rosemary oil has been associated with improved cognitive function. Inhaling its aroma is believed to stimulate mental clarity, enhance focus, and promote alertness. This quality makes it a popular choice for aromatherapy during periods of studying or work.

Mood Enhancement: Rosemary oil's aroma is known to have mood-lifting properties. Inhaling its scent can help alleviate feelings of stress, anxiety, and fatigue, creating a sense of relaxation and well-being.

Memory Support: As an extension of its historical reputation, rosemary oil is often linked to memory enhancement. Research suggests that the aroma of rosemary may have a positive impact on memory retention and cognitive performance.

Hair and Scalp Health: Rosemary oil is prized for its potential to promote hair growth and strengthen the hair shaft. It can be added to shampoos and conditioners to support a healthy scalp.

Respiratory Support: The oil's camphoraceous aroma can help open up the airways, making it a useful aid for relieving respiratory congestion and discomfort.

Pain Relief: Rosemary oil's anti-inflammatory properties make it a valuable tool for alleviating muscle pain, joint discomfort, and headaches. When diluted and massaged onto the skin, it can provide relief from tension and soreness.

Digestive Wellness: Rosemary oil can aid digestion by promoting the production of digestive enzymes. Inhaling its scent or using it in massage blends can help alleviate digestive discomfort.

Skin Revitalization: The oil's antioxidants contribute to its potential in promoting skin health by protecting against free radicals. It can be used topically to rejuvenate the skin and reduce the appearance of wrinkles.

Balancing Tradition with Science:

Rosemary oil's historical significance is fortified by modern research that validates its therapeutic effects. Its journey through time exemplifies its continued relevance in contemporary wellness practices.

Conclusion:

Rosemary oil's odyssey from ancient rituals to modern wellness routines is a testament to its enduring allure and multifaceted potential. Whether utilized for cognitive enhancement, physical relief, or beautification, rosemary oil offers an aromatic embrace of nature's wisdom. In the fragrant leaves of the rosemary plant, we find a reminder of nature's ability to invigorate, uplift, and fortify. Through rosemary oil, we embrace the vitality and clarity that nature bestows upon us, inviting these qualities into our lives and fostering a sense of rejuvenation and balance.

Chapter Twelve:

Thyme Oil: A Potent Essence of Wellness and Vigor

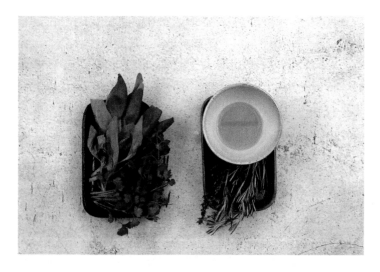

"As time flows, thyme oil remains, a timeless essence of nature's healing embrace." - Hippocrates

In the world of essential oils, thyme oil stands as a potent and versatile elixir of health and vitality. Derived from the tiny aromatic leaves and flowering tops of the evergreen thyme plant (Thymus vulgaris) this oil has traversed cultures and generations, earning its reputation as a natural remedy and aromatic treasure.

With its unique fragrance, versatile properties, and potential health benefits, thyme oil has earned its place as a cherished component of aromatherapy, traditional medicine, and even modern wellness practices.

Historical Significance and Cultural Uses

The use of thyme for medicinal purposes can be traced back to ancient civilizations such as the Egyptians, Greeks, and Romans. Thyme was revered for its antimicrobial and antiseptic properties, and its dried leaves were often used as incense to purify the air and protect against infections. The aromatic qualities of thyme made it a favored component in perfumes, cosmetics, and embalming practices.

Greek and Roman soldiers were known to take baths infused with thyme before battles, believing it would provide courage and strength. Ancient medical texts, including the works of Hippocrates and Dioscorides, documented thyme's therapeutic applications for respiratory issues, digestive problems, and wound healing.

Chemical Composition and Therapeutic Properties

Thyme oil owes its potent properties to its rich composition of bioactive compounds, including thymol, carvacrol, linalool, and terpinene-4-ol. Thymol, in particular, is renowned for its antimicrobial properties and is commonly used in modern mouthwashes and disinfectants. Carvacrol exhibits antifungal and antibacterial effects, while linalool contributes to thyme oil's calming and relaxing properties.

These components collectively make thyme oil a multifaceted remedy, with potential benefits ranging from supporting respiratory health to promoting relaxation and soothing sore muscles.

In aromatherapy, it is used to boost energy, uplift the mood, and provide mental clarity. The oil's aromatic presence can infuse spaces with a sense of renewal and vigor, making it a valuable tool for combating mental fatigue and lethargy.

A Multifaceted Arsenal:

Thyme oil's versatile applications span across several aspects of health and wellness:

Immune Support: Thyme oil is celebrated for its potential to bolster the immune system. Its antimicrobial properties make it a natural defense against bacteria, viruses, and fungal infections.

Respiratory Relief: The oil's expectorant qualities can provide relief from respiratory congestion and discomfort. Inhaling thyme oil vapor or using it in steam inhalation can help clear the airways.

Muscle Relaxation: Thyme oil's analgesic properties make it effective for reducing muscle pain and tension. When diluted and massaged onto the skin, it can provide relief from soreness and discomfort.

Digestive Aid: Thyme oil's carminative properties can aid in digestion by reducing bloating, gas, and indigestion. It can also stimulate the appetite.

Skin Health: Thyme oil's antibacterial and antifungal attributes make it useful for skin care. It can help alleviate acne, eczema, and other skin irritations.

Stress Relief: The soothing aroma of thyme oil can have a calming effect on the mind and body. Incorporating thyme oil into relaxation rituals, massages, or baths can help reduce stress and anxiety.

Aromatherapy Diffusion: Adding a few drops of thyme oil to an essential oil diffuser can create an invigorating and uplifting ambiance in your living space. It's especially beneficial during seasons when respiratory concerns are prevalent.

DIY Cleaning Solutions: Harness thyme oil's natural antibacterial properties by adding it to homemade cleaning solutions. It can help disinfect surfaces while leaving a refreshing scent.

Precautions and Guidelines:

Pregnancy and Nursing: Pregnant women and nursing mothers should avoid using thyme oil, as it may stimulate contractions and affect hormonal balance.

Epilepsy: Individuals with epilepsy should use thyme oil cautiously, as it may trigger seizures due to its high camphor content.

A Bridge Between Tradition and Modernity:

Thyme oil's historical significance is reinforced by scientific research that confirms its therapeutic effects. Its journey through time speaks to its enduring value and relevance.

Conclusion:

Thyme oil's passage from ancient remedies to contemporary wellness practices is a testament to its robust and enduring qualities. Whether employed for its immune-boosting power, respiratory relief, or mental invigoration, thyme oil presents an aromatic tapestry of health and vitality. Adhering to guidelines and precautions ensures its safe and effective use. Through thyme oil, we connect with the resilience and vigor that nature offers us, inviting these qualities into our lives and fostering a sense of well-being and strength. In the aromatic embrace of thyme oil, we find a reminder of nature's capacity to fortify, protect, and rejuvenate both body and spirit.

Chapter Thirteen:

Clove Oil: The Aromatic Jewel of Wellness and Tradition

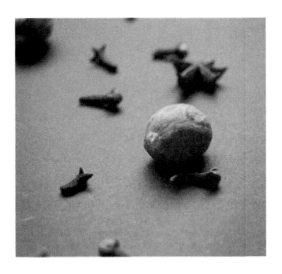

"In every drop of clove oil, the essence of eons past, preserving its place in modern healing."
-Deepak Chopra

A mong the vast array of essential oils, clove oil stands as a treasured jewel, renowned for its rich history, distinctive aroma, and numerous health benefits. Derived from the dried flower buds of the clove tree (Syzygium aromaticum), clove oil has been revered for centuries for its potent therapeutic properties and versatile applications. From ancient civilizations to modern holistic practices, clove oil continues to captivate with its aromatic allure and wellness offerings. This article delves into the history, uses, benefits, and precautions associated with clove oil, illuminating its multifaceted nature as a natural remedy and aromatic delight.

Botanical Heritage and Ancient Wisdom:

The journey of clove oil begins with the clove tree, native to the Moluccas (Spice Islands) in Indonesia. This evergreen tree produces small, nail-shaped flower buds that, once dried, are used to extract the aromatic oil. These buds have been a coveted commodity since antiquity, drawing traders and explorers from distant lands to the source of their aromatic treasure.

Cultural Significance and Historical Elegance:

Clove's cultural significance spans civilizations and epochs. Ancient Chinese and Indian civilizations used cloves for medicinal and culinary purposes, while in ancient Egypt, they were employed as a breath freshener. The Greeks and Romans embraced cloves for their aromatic qualities, and they became an integral part of Middle Eastern perfumes. In medieval Europe, cloves symbolized luxury and were highly valued not only for their flavor and fragrance but also for their reputed medicinal prowess.

Aromatic Enchantment and Therapeutic Touch:

Clove oil's aroma is intense, warm, and spicy, with undertones of sweetness and earthiness. This distinctive scent is the result of its main component, eugenol, which contributes to the oil's therapeutic properties. In aromatherapy, the aroma of clove oil is believed to uplift the spirit, promote mental clarity, and provide a sense of comfort.

A Pantheon of Health Benefits:

Clove oil's multifaceted health benefits span a wide spectrum:

Oral Health: Clove oil has been celebrated for its role in oral care for centuries. Its antimicrobial properties can help combat bacteria responsible for bad breath and dental issues. It's often found in toothpaste, mouthwash, and oral hygiene products.

Digestive Comfort: Clove oil can support healthy digestion by promoting the production of digestive enzymes. Its carminative properties can alleviate symptoms of indigestion, bloating, and gas.

Pain Relief: Clove oil's analgesic and anti-inflammatory qualities make it an effective remedy for relieving muscle and joint pain. It's often used in massage blends or diluted with a carrier oil for topical application.

Respiratory Support: Inhaling the vapors of clove oil can provide relief from respiratory congestion and discomfort due to its expectorant properties.

Antioxidant Power: The high antioxidant content of clove oil contributes to its potential to combat oxidative stress and free radical damage, thereby supporting overall health.

A Fusion of Tradition and Modern Science:

Clove oil's rich historical tapestry is interwoven with modern scientific research that validates its therapeutic attributes. Its journey through time exemplifies its enduring significance and value in modern wellness practices.

Conclusion:

Clove oil's passage from ancient traditions to contemporary wellness routines is a testament to its enduring appeal and multi faceted potential. Whether utilized for oral care, pain relief, or respiratory support, clove oil offers an aromatic embrace of nature's wisdom. Adhering to guidelines and precautions ensures its safe and effective use. Through clove oil, we connect with the historical significance and healing potency that nature offers us, inviting these qualities into our lives and fostering a sense of well-being, tradition, and vibrancy. In the aromatic depths of clove oil, we find a reminder of nature's ability to comfort, heal, and empower both the body and spirit

Chapter Fourteen:

Crafting Remedies: Practical Applications of Essential Oils

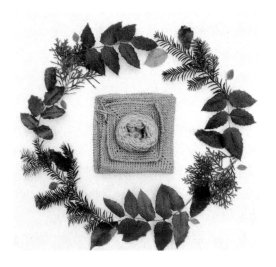

The heart of the book unfolds in this chapter where theory meets practice. Here, we delve into the art of crafting remedies using essential oils for a multitude of first aid scenarios. Whether it's soothing minor burns, alleviating headaches, or aiding digestion, each section provides step-by-step instructions to create safe and effective blends. With an emphasis on proper dilution and application techniques, readers are empowered to harness the healing potential of essential oils with confidence.

Notes: Although the following blends use a combination of the ten essential oils described in the previous chapters, there are some which use other oils as well.
Usual mix is 4-10 drops in 10ml of base oil
Never use directly on the skin unless otherwise instructed
Start with a small test area

ANTI BACTERIAL SURFACE SPRAY:

10 drops clove oil

10 drops citronella oil

5 drops tea tree oil

1 cup distilled water

Combine in a spray bottle for a natural and aromatic antibacterial room and surface spray.

ATHLETE'S FOOT (FUNGUS INFECTION):

Tea tree oil is an excellent choice and combined as follows and applied daily will kill the infection causing athlete's foot. Ensure that good foot hygiene is maintained and try to avoid the overwearing of sweaty trainers.

10 drops tea tree oil

10 drops eucalyptus oil

in 10ml of a light base oil like grape seed. Use twice a day.

BLISTERS:

Apply a few drops of lavender oil and chamomile oil to a plaster and cover the blister. Try not to pop the blister but when it does, use tea tree oil to disinfect and prevent infection.

BOILS:

Apply a hot compress with 2 drops of thyme oil. Once the boil has burst, apply a dressing with lavender oil and tea tree oil. Change the dressing daily.

BRUISES:

Apply lavender oil directly to the area and massage frequently with arnica. Witch hazel applied to the bruise will also help.

BURNS (HOT WATER ETC):

Lavender oil is the perfect oil to apply to burnt skin to promote healing. First aid for burns is always plenty of cold water to the area, but once the stinging feeling has passed then lavender oil can be applied. A couple of drops of tea tree oil in the mix will act as a disinfectant as well.

COLDS AND COUGHS:

   4 drops tea tree oil

   5 drops eucalyptus oil

   4 drops lavender oil

blended together and put into a diffuser in the bedroom at night will help with breathing.

You can also put a drop or two on a tissue and inhale the vapors.

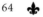
A room spray of 5 drops of thyme oil in water will act as an antiseptic. You can add 4 drops lavender oil to help with sleep as well.

4 drops eucalyptus oil
4 drops peppermint oil

in 10ml of a carrier oil. Massage back and chest three to four times a day.

3 drops thyme oil
3 drops rosemary oil (to reduce respiratory inflammation)

in 10ml carrier oil. Use as a back rub three times a day.

3 drops ginger (warming)
3 drops lemon (antiseptic)

in 10ml carrier oil. This will help ease congestion and reduce coughing. Rub onto the chest and back three times a day.

Respiratory Support Blend:
3 drops clove oil

3 drops peppermint oil

2 drops eucalyptus oil

2 drops tea tree oil

Diffuse or use in a steam inhalation for respiratory relief. Use as often as required.

WHOOPING COUGH:

Put 5 drops of thyme oil in steaming water and inhale the vapors three times a day.

COLD SORES:

Put 1 drop of tea tree oil (antiviral) and 1 drop of geranium oil (anti-inflammatory) on a cotton bud and apply directly to the cold sore.

> 2 drops peppermint oil
>
> 2 drops lavender oil

in 5ml base oil. Apply frequently to the cold sore.

EARACHE:

Add 2 drops lavender oil to 5ml of warmed almond oil. After soaking some cotton wool in this, plug the earhole. Change twice a day. If any pus is being produced, it's important to get it checked by a doctor.

GUM DISEASE:

> 2 drops tea tree oil
>
> 2 drops thyme oil

in 10ml water and rinse mouth out two to three times a day. Do not swallow.

HAIR AND SCALP TREATMENT:

> 5 drops tea tree oil
>
> 4 drops rosemary oil
>
> 2 drops peppermint oil
>
> 1 drop lavender oil

Add to 10ml carrier oil and massage daily into the scalp to promote a healthy scalp and hair.

If available, add 3 drops of cedar wood oil to the blend; this is very nourishing and will give it a wonderful fragrance.

Another one:

6 drops rosemary oil

4 drops lavender oil

2 drops thyme oil

1 drop geranium oil

Mix with 20ml carrier oil and apply to the scalp daily to support hair growth and maintain scalp health.

HEADACHE:

3 drops peppermint oil

2 drops lavender oil

in 10ml base oil. Rub on temples when required.

Relaxing mix for tension headaches

2 drops chamomile oil

3 drops rosemary oil

in 10ml of base oil. Rub on temples whenever needed.

Sinus Headaches:

Put a few drops of eucalyptus oil into hot water and inhale the vapor.

Pms Headache:

2 drops geranium oil

3 drops lavender oil

in 10ml base oil. Rub on temples

IMMUNE-BOOSTING BLEND:

4 drops clove oil

3 drops citronella oil

2 drops eucalyptus oil

2 drops rosemary oil

Dilute with 20ml carrier oil before applying to the skin or using in a diffuser.

INDIGESTION AND RELATED PROBLEMS:

Peppermint oil is the ideal oil for indigestion and while it is not recommended that you ingest essential oils, you will find peppermint oil in many pharmaceutical preparations for indigestion. Just two drops in some warm water, sipped slowly, will work wonders.

Chamomile oil will help soothe a sore stomach with its calming and relaxing properties when diluted with a carrier and rubbed on the abdomen. It's recommended you rub in a clockwise direction.

Lavender oil will help if the stomach upset is due to stress.

Ginger oil is good for relieving nausea and vomiting. Dilute in a carrier oil and then gently rub on the abdomen.

Cardamom oil is a carminative and relieves gas and bloating of the stomach. Dilute in a carrier oil and then gently rub on the abdomen.

INSECT BITES:

2 drops eucalyptus oil

2 drops lavender oil

2 drops tea tree oil

in 10ml carrier oil. Apply three or four times a day.

A lovely cooling combination is:

3 drops peppermint oil

2 drops tea tree oil

in 10ml carrier oil when needed.

Insect Repellent:

Citronella oil can be used neat but it is strongly advised you do a patch test first. Otherwise mix 10 drops in 10ml of carrier oil and apply to exposed skin. Both eucalyptus oil and lavender oil can be added to this blend.

CITRONELLA CANDLE BLEND

20 drops citronella oil

5 drops lavender oil

5 drops eucalyptus oil

Mix these oils with melted soy wax to create your own bug-repelling citronella candles.

Lice Infestation:

Add 10 drops tea tree oil to your shampoo, lather it up and leave for about ten minutes before rinsing. Do this daily for a week. Also add 10 drops to a hair conditioner; apply to the hair and, using a nit comb, comb the hair through to remove the eggs which attach to the hair.

Muscle Aches and Pains:

5 drops lavender oil

5 drops peppermint oil

in 10ml base oil. Massage twice a day.

5 drops rosemary oil

5 drops chamomile oil

in 10ml base oil. Massage twice a day.

>   4 drops clove oil

>   3 drops marjoram oil

>   2 drops ginger oil

>   1 drop lavender oil

Dilute with a carrier oil and use for massage on areas of discomfort.

Massaging with either one of these will relieve aching muscles, especially after exercise.

NAUSEA AND TRAVEL SICKNESS:

Try inhaling a few drops of peppermint oil and citronella oil on a tissue.

RING WORM (FUNGAL INFECTION)

>   3 drops tea tree oil

>   3 drops thyme oil

in 5ml carrier oil. Apply to the area twice a day. Keep using it for at least ten days after the infection has gone.

SKIN PROBLEMS:

DRY SKIN

There are many oils that will help with dry and flaky skin. Rose oil is probably the most useful. It is very expensive but a lovely oil to use if you can afford it.

It is a good idea to do a patch test, especially if the blend is being used on the face.

>   3 drops chamomile oil

>   3 drops lavender oil

in 10ml carrier oil. Use daily.

> 4 drops lavender oil
>
> 3 drops geranium oil

in 10ml carrier oil. Use daily.

…and a very luxurious one…

> 2 drops rose oil
>
> 2 drops ylang ylang oil
>
> 2 drops chamomile oil

in 10ml carrier oil. Use daily.

Carrot oil is a very nourishing oil for the skin. Combine it with the lovely scent of jasmine oil in a carrier oil.

SUNBURNT SKIN

> 2 drops lavender oil
>
> 2 drops chamomile oil

in 10ml almond oil. Apply to unbroken skin three or four times a day.

SKIN SOOTHING BLEND

> 5 drops tea tree oil
>
> 4 drops lavender oil
>
> 3 drops chamomile oil
>
> 1 drop geranium oil

Dilute with 20ml carrier oil and apply to irritated skin for soothing relief.

SLEEP:

There are many oils which can be used for helping you sleep. The first two mixes use the oils listed above; the other mixes use different oils which have been shown to help.

They can be massaged onto the skin or used in a diffuser. If you haven't got a diffuser, simply dropping the oils into hot water will release the vapors to inhale.

Skin mix (rub on temples/upper arms and chest before bed)
    2 drops lavender oil

    2 drops chamomile oil

    2 drops geranium oil

in 10ml base oil.

    2 drops rosemary oil

    3 drops chamomile oil

in 10ml base oil.

Use these other wonderful oils in a container of hot, steamy water next to your bed.

    3 drops bergamot oil (lowers your blood pressure and heart rate)

    3 drops cedar wood oil (calming and relaxing)

    2 drops vetivert oil (has an earthy smell to ground and slow your thoughts)

    2 drops bergamot oil

    2 drops marjoram oil (has a sweet fragrance to quieten your thoughts)

    2 drops clary sage oil (known to help with depression and raise your spirits)

    3 drops chamomile oil

    4 drops lavender oil

in 10ml carrier oil.

Throat Infection

Add 10 drops of tea tree oil to a glass of warm water and gargle with the mixture three to four times a day.

Toothache

Apply a drop of clove oil to an ear bud and place carefully on affected tooth. This will relieve pain until you can see a dentist.

Using a warm compress on the cheek next to the sore tooth may help. Make one using a few drops of chamomile oil and lavender oil. Put onto a wad of cotton wool and apply to the area.

Conclusion

As we conclude our exploration, readers are invited to broaden their perspective and embrace a holistic approach to well-being. Essential oils, as we've discovered, are not isolated remedies but conduits to a deeper connection with ourselves and nature. Mindfulness practices, meditation, and self-care rituals are enhanced by the inclusion of these oils. This book serves as a reminder that first aid is not merely about addressing physical ailments—it's about nurturing our entire being

In *Essential Oils for First Aid: A Comprehensive Aromatherapy Guide to Healing*, we embarked on a journey that transcends time, bridging ancient wisdom with modern science. As the world seeks solace in nature's embrace, this book serves as a guiding light, illuminating the path toward a more holistic and harmonious way of tending to our well-being. So, with an open heart and a curious mind, step into the aromatic world of essential oils and discover the transformative power they hold within their fragrant drops.

Thank you for reading this book, I have enjoyed writing it and would appreciate you writing a review with your thoughts and comments.

Printed in Great Britain
by Amazon

40189318R00046